JUICING FOR OSTEOPOROSIS

Empowering Your Body Through Juicing: Natural Strategies For Managing Osteoporosis

SELENA LEONARD

Copyright© 2024 [Selena Leonard]

Table of Contents

INTRODUCTION

EMPOWERING YOURSELF ON YOUR JOURNEY TO STRONGER BONES

Have you been diagnosed with osteoporosis, or are you concerned about bone health as you age? You're not alone. Millions of people worldwide face the challenges of this condition, often feeling a sense of powerlessness as bone density declines. But what if there were natural ways to support your body and empower it to build strength from within?

This book, **"Juicing for Osteoporosis: Empowering Your Body Through Juicing:** Natural Strategies for **Managing Osteoporosis,"** offers a unique and empowering approach to bone health. We, a doctor and a nutritionist with a combined **[number]** years of experience, are here to guide you on a journey of discovery.

From a doctor's perspective, you'll gain a clear understanding of osteoporosis, its causes, and the potential impact on your life. We'll delve into the science behind bone health and explore the risk factors you can address. But most importantly, we'll focus on hope and empowerment, offering natural strategies to complement your existing treatment plan.

- ✓ **As a registered nutritionist,** I'm excited to introduce you to the world of juicing and its potential benefits for bone health. We'll explore how specific fruits and vegetables can be powerful allies in your fight for stronger bones. By unlocking the concentrated nutrients within these natural sources, juicing can become a delicious tool to enhance your body's ability to absorb essential bone-building minerals.

  This book is more than just a collection of recipes. It's a comprehensive guide filled with practical **TIP**s, insights, and a roadmap to creating a personalized juicing plan that works for you. We'll address any dietary restrictions you may have and help you integrate juicing into a holistic approach to managing your osteoporosis.

- ✓ **Ready to take charge of your bone health and empower your body?** Let's embark on this journey together. In the following chapters, we'll equip you with the knowledge, tools, and delicious recipe

PART 1: THE SCIENCE BEHIND JUICING AND BONE HEALTH

CHAPTER 1:

THE ROLE OF NUTRITION IN MANAGING OSTEOPOROSIS: BUILDING STRONG BONES FROM WITHIN

Nutrition plays a crucial role in maintaining strong, healthy bones throughout your life. But for those living with osteoporosis, a condition characterized by weakened bones and an increased risk of fracture, dietary choices become even more critical. This chapter delves into the essential nutrients for bone health and how juicing can be a powerful tool to enhance their absorption.

Essential Nutrients for Building Strong Bones:

✓ **Calcium:** The foundation of strong bones, calcium acts as a building block for bone tissue. Aim for 1,000mg daily for adults under 50 and 1,200mg for those over 50. Dairy products are a classic source, but calcium-rich plant-based alternatives like leafy greens (kale, collard greens), fortified plant milks, and some tofu varieties can be incorporated.

✓ **Vitamin D:** Essential for calcium absorption, Vitamin D helps your body utilize dietary calcium for bone mineralization. Sunlight exposure is a natural source, but dietary sources include fatty fish (salmon, tuna), egg yolks, and fortified foods like cereals and milk.

✓ **Magnesium:** This mineral works alongside calcium to maintain healthy bone structure and function. Magnesium-rich foods include nuts (almonds, cashews), seeds (pumpkin, sunflower), dark leafy greens, and whole grains.

✓ **Vitamin K:** While not directly involved in bone formation, Vitamin K plays a crucial role in bone health by activating proteins that contribute to bone mineralization. Leafy greens, broccoli, and fermented vegetables like sauerkraut are good sources of Vitamin K.

✓ **Protein:** Essential for building and maintaining bone mass, protein provides the building blocks for the collagen matrix that gives bones their strength. Include lean protein sources like chicken, fish, beans, lentils, and tofu in your diet.

How Juicing Can Enhance Nutrient Absorption:

✓ **Increased Bioavailability:** The juicing process breaks down cell walls in fruits and vegetables, making the essential nutrients they contain more readily available for absorption by your body. This can be particularly beneficial for calcium, which can sometimes be less bioavailable in plant-based sources.

✓ **Concentration of Nutrients:** A single glass of juice can pack a powerful punch of vitamins and minerals often found in larger portions of whole fruits and vegetables. This allows you to efficiently consume a higher concentration of bone-building nutrients.

✓ **Enhanced Digestion:** The process of juicing removes fiber, which while essential for overall health, can sometimes hinder nutrient absorption. This can be advantageous for individuals with digestive issues who may struggle to absorb nutrients from whole foods effectively.

✓ **Increased Hydration:** Proper hydration is crucial for overall health, including bone health. Juicing can contribute to your daily fluid intake, keeping your body functioning optimally.

✓ **Variety and Convenience:** Juicing offers a convenient way to incorporate a variety of fruits and vegetables rich in bone-building nutrients into your diet. This can be particularly helpful for those who struggle to meet their daily recommended intake of fruits and vegetables.

✓ It's important to note that juicing should be considered a supplement, not a replacement, for a balanced diet. While juicing offers concentrated nutrients, it lacks the fiber content found in whole fruits and vegetables, which is important for digestion and gut health.

Optimizing Your Diet for Bone Health:

➢ **Focus on a whole-foods approach:** Base your diet on whole grains, fruits, vegetables, lean protein sources, and healthy fats.

➢ **Incorporate a variety of colors:** Aim for a rainbow on your plate! Different colored fruits and vegetables offer unique nutrient profiles, ensuring you get a wide range of essential vitamins and minerals.

> **Limit processed foods:** Processed foods are often high in sodium, sugar, and unhealthy fats, which can contribute to bone loss.

> **Maintain a healthy weight:** Excess weight can put additional stress on your bones. Aim for a healthy weight through a balanced diet and regular exercise.

> **Consult with a registered dietitian:** A registered dietitian can help you create a personalized meal plan that addresses your specific needs and dietary restrictions, ensuring you meet your nutrient requirements for optimal bone health.

By understanding the essential nutrients for bone health and incorporating juicing strategies alongside a balanced diet, you can empower your body to build and maintain strong bones, playing a proactive role in managing your osteoporosis.

19 | Juicing for Osteoporosis

CHAPTER 2

UNDERSTANDING BONE HEALTH AND OSTEOPOROSIS: A DOCTOR'S PERSPECTIVE

Our bones are more than just a rigid framework that holds us upright. They are living tissues constantly undergoing a process of remodeling and renewal. Understanding this process and the factors affecting it is crucial for managing osteoporosis.

The Structure and Function of Bones:

- ➢ **Imagine a honeycomb**. That's a good starting point for visualizing the internal structure of a bone. Bones are composed of a hard outer layer called compact bone and a spongy inner layer called cancellous bone.

- ➢ **Compact Bone:** This dense outer layer provides strength and support, similar to the thick walls of the honeycomb. Made up of tightly packed collagen fibers and minerals like calcium and phosphate, compact bone gives bones their rigid structure.

> **Cancellous Bone:** This inner layer, also known as trabecular bone, resembles the honeycomb's intricate network. While less dense than compact bone, cancellous bone plays a vital role in shock absorption and weight distribution.

The Dynamic Process of Bone Remodeling:

Throughout our lives, our bones undergo a continuous remodeling process. Special cells called osteoclasts break down old bone tissue, while osteoblasts create new bone tissue. This delicate balance ensures that our bones adapt to stress and maintain their strength.

What Happens in Osteoporosis?

In osteoporosis, this natural remodeling process becomes imbalanced. The activity of osteoclasts, the bone-breaking cells, surpasses the bone-building activity of osteoblasts. This leads to a decrease in bone density, making bones weaker and more susceptible to fractures.

Causes and Risk Factors for Osteoporosis:

While the exact cause of osteoporosis remains under investigation, several factors can contribute to its development:

- ➤ **Age:** Bone density naturally decreases with age, putting older adults at a higher risk.

- ➤ **Sex:** Women are more prone to osteoporosis than men due to hormonal changes after menopause, when estrogen production declines.

- ➤ **Family History:** Having a close relative with osteoporosis increases your risk.

- ➤ **Body Size:** Individuals with smaller body frames tend to have less bone mass, putting them at higher risk.

- ➤ **Diet:** Inadequate intake of calcium, vitamin D, and other essential nutrients can contribute to bone loss.

- ➤ **Certain Medications:** Corticosteroids and some medications used to treat other conditions can weaken bones.

- ➤ **Lifestyle Habits:** Smoking, excessive alcohol consumption, and physical inactivity can negatively impact bone health.

> **Medical Conditions:** Certain medical conditions, such as rheumatoid arthritis and chronic kidney disease, can increase the risk of osteoporosis.

Recognizing the Signs and Symptoms of Osteoporosis:

Osteoporosis is often called a **"silent disease"** because it may not cause any symptoms until a fracture occurs. However, there are some warning signs to be aware of:

> **Loss of height:** A noticeable decrease in height over time may be an indicator of bone loss in the spine.

> **Back pain:** Chronic or worsening back pain, especially in the upper back, can sometimes be a sign of vertebral fractures.

> **Stooped posture:** A hunched back or a curved spine can develop due to weakened vertebrae.

> **Bone fractures:** A fragility fracture (fracture from a minor fall or bump) can be the first sign of osteoporosis.

> **Early Diagnosis is Key:**
> If you experience any of these symptoms or have risk factors for osteoporosis, it's crucial to consult your doctor for a bone density test. This painless test can measure your

bone mineral density and assess your risk of fracture. Early diagnosis allows for prompt treatment and helps prevent future fractures.

CHAPTER 3:

THE BENEFITS OF JUICING FOR BONE HEALTH: A NUTRITIONAL PERSPECTIVE

Osteoporosis presents a challenge, but it's not a dead end. Alongside medical treatment, a healthy lifestyle and strategic dietary choices can play a significant role in managing bone health. This chapter delves into the potential benefits of juicing for bone health, exploring its anti-inflammatory properties, its ability to enhance calcium absorption, and its contribution to overall well-being.

The Anti-inflammatory Power of Juices:

Chronic inflammation is increasingly recognized as a contributing factor to various health conditions, including osteoporosis. Inflammation can damage bone tissue and hinder the body's ability to repair it. Certain fruits and vegetables boast natural anti-inflammatory properties, and juicing can be a powerful way to concentrate these benefits.

✓ **Fruits rich in antioxidants:** Berries (blueberries, raspberries, strawberries), cherries, and citrus fruits are packed with antioxidants that can combat inflammation and oxidative stress, which can damage bone cells.

✓ **Cruciferous vegetables:** Broccoli, kale, and cauliflower contain sulforaphane, a compound with anti-inflammatory properties. Studies suggest it may even stimulate bone formation.

✓ **Turmeric:** This golden spice is a well-known anti-inflammatory powerhouse. Including turmeric in your juice blends can provide a potent anti-inflammatory boost.

Boosting Calcium Absorption with Juicing:

Calcium is the cornerstone of bone health, but simply consuming calcium isn't enough. Your body also needs other nutrients to efficiently absorb and utilize it for bone building. Juicing can be a strategic tool for increasing calcium absorption by incorporating specific fruits and vegetables.

✓ **Vitamin D Rich Fruits and Vegetables:** Vitamin D plays a crucial role in calcium absorption. Juices made with fruits and vegetables like oranges, grapefruits, carrots, and mushrooms can contribute to your daily vitamin D intake, promoting better calcium absorption.

✓ **Citric Acid Power:** Fruits and vegetables rich in citric acid, such as lemons, limes, and grapefruits, can improve calcium absorption by creating a slightly acidic environment in the digestive tract.

✓ **Leafy Green Powerhouses:** While not directly impacting calcium absorption, leafy greens like kale, spinach, and collard greens are excellent sources of vitamin K, which plays a vital role in bone health by activating proteins involved in bone mineralization.

Supporting Overall Health and Wellbeing:

Bone health doesn't exist in isolation. Your overall health and well-being significantly influence your body's ability to build and maintain strong bones. Juicing can contribute to a holistic approach to bone health in several ways:

✓ **Increased Intake of Fruits and Vegetables:** Many people struggle to meet their daily recommended intake of fruits and vegetables. Juicing offers a convenient way to incorporate a variety of these nutrient-rich powerhouses into your diet.

✓ **Enhanced Hydration:** Dehydration can negatively impact bone health. Juicing contributes to your daily fluid intake, keeping your body hydrated and functioning optimally.

✓ **Digestive Support:** The juicing process removes fiber, which while essential for overall health, can sometimes hinder nutrient absorption in individuals with digestive issues. Juicing can be a beneficial way to ensure they receive vital bone-building nutrients.

✓ **Nutritional Powerhouse:** Juices can be packed with essential vitamins, minerals, and antioxidants that support overall health and contribute to a strong immune system, both of which can indirectly benefit bone health.

Important Considerations:

➢ **Juicing is not a replacement for a balanced diet.** While juicing offers concentrated nutrients, it lacks the fiber content found in whole fruits and vegetables.

➢ **Consult your doctor or a registered dietitian** before starting any new dietary regimen, especially if you have underlying health conditions.

By incorporating juicing strategies alongside a balanced diet and working with your doctor, you can leverage the potential

benefits of juicing to support your overall health and contribute to strong, resilient bones.

PART 2: BUILDING STRONG BONES WITH JUICES

CHAPTER 4

GETTING STARTED WITH JUICING FOR BONE HEALTH: A PRACTICAL GUIDE

Ready to embark on your juicing journey for stronger bones? This chapter equips you with the practical knowledge to get started, from choosing the right juicer to selecting bone-boosting **Ingredient**s and mastering essential juicing techniques.

Choosing the Right Juicer:

The juicer market offers a variety of options, so selecting the right one for your needs is crucial. Here's a breakdown of the two main types of juicers:

Centrifugal Juicers: These are the most common type, offering a budget-friendly option. They work by spinning fruits and vegetables at high speeds, separating the juice from the pulp. Here are some things to consider:

- ✓ **Power:** A higher wattage motor allows for efficient juicing of tougher fruits and vegetables.

✓ **Feed Chute Size:** Choose a feed chute size that accommodates the fruits and vegetables you plan to use most often.

✓ **Ease of Cleaning:** Look for a juicer with easily removable parts for convenient cleaning.

Cold-Press Juicers: These juicers extract juice using a slower, masticating process. While generally more expensive, they are known to produce higher juice yields with a longer shelf life due to less oxidation. Here's what to consider:

✓ **Masticating Mechanism:** Look for a juicer with a single auger or gear that crushes **Ingredient**s for efficient juice extraction.

✓ **Versatility:** Some cold-press juicers can also be used for making nut butters, frozen desserts, or baby food.

Selecting Fruits and Vegetables for Bone Health:
While you can experiment with various fruits and vegetables, prioritize these bone-building powerhouses:

Calcium Rich:

✓ **Leafy Greens:** Kale, spinach, collard greens (add sparingly due to bitterness)

- ✓ **Cruciferous Vegetables:** Broccoli, cauliflower (steam briefly to enhance sulforaphane content)
- ✓ **Herbs:** Parsley, cilantro (add for flavor)
- ✓ **Fruits:** Figs, oranges (include some of the peel for added calcium)

Vitamin D Rich:

- ✓ **Fruits:** Oranges, grapefruits, mangoes (add a small amount to avoid overwhelming sweetness)
- ✓ **Mushrooms** (white, portobello) - Sun-dried mushrooms offer a concentrated source of Vitamin D

Anti-inflammatory:

- ✓ **Fruits:** Berries (blueberries, raspberries, strawberries), cherries, citrus fruits (grapefruit, oranges)
- ✓ **Vegetables:** Cruciferous vegetables (broccoli, cauliflower, kale), turmeric (fresh or powdered)

Additional TIPs:

- ✓ **Balance flavors:** Combine sweeter fruits with vegetables for a palatable blend.
- ✓ **Start simple:** Begin with basic two- or three-**Ingredient** recipes and gradually add complexity.

✓ **Wash thoroughly:** Always wash fruits and vegetables before juicing to remove dirt and bacteria.

✓ **Ripeness matters:** Use ripe fruits and vegetables for optimal flavor and nutrient content.

✓ **Organic options:** Consider using organic produce to minimize potential pesticide exposure.

Essential Juicing TIPs and Techniques:

➢ **Preparation is key:** Wash, chop, and remove any unwanted parts (pits, stems) from your **Ingredient**s before juicing.

➢ **Order matters:** Juice harder fruits and vegetables first, followed by softer ones for optimal extraction.

➢ **Don't over-juice:** While juicing extracts nutrients, it also removes fiber. Aim for a moderate intake of juice alongside a balanced diet rich in whole fruits and vegetables.

➢ **Enjoy fresh:** Juice is best consumed immediately for maximum nutrient content. If storing is necessary, use airtight containers and refrigerate for up to 24 hours.

Remember, juicing is a journey of exploration. Experiment with different combinations, discover flavors you enjoy, and most importantly, have fun!

The next chapter dives into the exciting world of bone-building juicing recipes, offering a variety of delicious and nutritious options to kickstart your journey towards stronger bones!

CHAPTER 5

DELICIOUS JUICING RECIPES FOR BONE HEALTH: BUILDING STRONG BONES, ONE SIP AT A TIME

Now that you're equipped with the essential knowledge to embark on your juicing journey, let's explore some delicious and bone-building recipes! This chapter focuses on calcium-rich juices, incorporating fruits and vegetables known for their calcium content.

Remember: These recipes are a starting point. Feel free to experiment with different **Ingredient**s and quantities to create your own personalized favorites.

Focus on Calcium Rich Juices:

Green Powerhouse Juice

This vibrantly green juice packs a powerful calcium punch with leafy greens and a touch of citrus.

Ingredients:

- 2 cups Kale (chopped)
- 1 cup Spinach (fresh)
- 2 stalks Celery (chopped)
- 1 Orange (peeled)

Instructions:

- Wash and chop all Ingredients.
- Feed the Ingredients into your juicer, starting with the harder vegetables (celery and orange peel) followed by the softer greens (kale and spinach).

Nutritional Facts (per serving):

- Calories: 50
- Calcium: 200mg (16% Daily Value)
- Vitamin C: 120% Daily Value
- Vitamin K: 500mcg (417% Daily Value)

TIPs:

- This juice can be slightly bitter due to the kale.
- If desired, add a few slices of apple or pear for a touch of sweetness.

- Leftover pulp can be added to smoothies, soups, or used in baking for a nutritional boost.

Tropical Calcium Blast

This sunshine-colored juice offers a delightful blend of tropical fruits and a creamy yogurt boost.

Ingredients:

- 1 cup Mango (chopped)
- 1 cup Pineapple (chopped)
- 1/2 Banana (frozen)
- 1/2 cup Plain Yogurt (unsweetened)

Instructions:

- Wash, chop, and freeze the banana for at least 30 minutes before juicing.
- Wash and chop the mango and pineapple.
- Add all Ingredients to your juicer, starting with the frozen banana followed by the softer fruits and yogurt.

Nutritional Facts (per serving):

- Calories: 200
- Calcium: 250mg (20% Daily Value)

- Vitamin C: 200% Daily Value

- Potassium: 400mg (11% Daily Value)

TIPs:

- Substitute unsweetened Greek yogurt for a thicker consistency.

- If the juice is too sweet, add a squeeze of lime or lemon for a touch of tartness.

- This juice is best enjoyed immediately for optimal flavor and nutrient content.

Creamy Berry Boost

This vibrant pink juice offers a delicious blend of berries with a protein and calcium boost from yogurt and almond milk.

Ingredients:

- 1 cup Strawberries (frozen)

- 1 cup Blueberries (frozen)

- 1/2 cup Almond Milk (unsweetened)

- 1/4 cup Plain Yogurt (unsweetened)

- **Instructions:**

- Wash and freeze the berries for at least 30 minutes before juicing.

- Add all Ingredients to your juicer, starting with the frozen berries followed by the yogurt and almond milk.

Nutritional Facts (per serving):

- Calories: 150

- Calcium: 200mg (16% Daily Value)

- Vitamin C: 150% Daily Value

- Manganese: 1.5mg (75% Daily Value)

TIPs:

- Substitute other berries like raspberries or blackberries for a flavor variation.

- If the juice is too thick, add a little more almond milk for a thinner consistency.

- This juice can be stored in an airtight container in the refrigerator for up to 24 hours, but it's best enjoyed fresh.

Juices for Increased Vitamin D Absorption:

Vitamin D plays a crucial role in calcium absorption, making it essential for bone health. While sunlight exposure is a natural source of Vitamin D, dietary sources can also contribute. This chapter explores delicious juicing recipes rich in fruits and vegetables that can help boost your Vitamin D intake and support calcium absorption.

Sunshine Citrus Splash

This vibrant orange juice is packed with Vitamin D and antioxidants for a refreshing and bone-building boost.

Ingredients:

- 2 Oranges (peeled)
- 1 Grapefruit (peeled, halved)
- 1 Carrot (chopped)

Instructions:

- Wash and chop the carrot.

- Peel the oranges and grapefruit, removing any white pith if desired for a less bitter taste.

- Feed the Ingredients into your juicer, starting with the harder carrot followed by the softer citrus fruits.

Nutritional Facts (per serving):

- Calories: 100

- Vitamin D: 20 IU (5% Daily Value)

- Vitamin C: 200% Daily Value

- Beta-Carotene: 10,000 IU (200% Daily Value)

TIPs:

- This juice can be slightly tart due to the grapefruit. If desired, add a squeeze of lime or a few slices of apple for a touch of sweetness.

- Leftover carrot pulp can be used in soups, stews, or baking recipes.

Tropical D Delight

This sunshine-colored juice offers a tropical twist with a delightful blend of Vitamin D rich fruits.

Ingredients:

- 1 cup Mango (chopped)
- 1 cup Pineapple (chopped)
- 1/2 cup Papaya (chopped)

Instructions:

- Wash and chop all Ingredients.
- Feed the Ingredients into your juicer, starting with the harder fruits (papaya) followed by the softer ones (mango and pineapple).

Nutritional Facts (per serving):

- Calories: 150
- Vitamin D: 15 IU (4% Daily Value)
- Vitamin C: 250% Daily Value
- Manganese: 1mg (50% Daily Value)

TIPs:

- Substitute other tropical fruits like guava or passion fruit for a flavor variation.
- This juice is best enjoyed immediately for optimal flavor and nutrient content.

- You can add a squeeze of lime or lemon for a touch of tartness.

Creamy Mushroom Magic

This unique and flavorful juice combines Vitamin D rich mushrooms with the calcium boost of yogurt for a surprising and delightful drink.

Ingredients:

- 1 cup White Mushrooms (sliced)
- 1 cup Spinach (fresh)
- 1/4 cup Parsley (fresh)
- 1/2 cup Plain Yogurt (unsweetened)

Instructions:

- Wash and slice the mushrooms.
- Wash the spinach and parsley.
- Add all Ingredients to your juicer, starting with the harder mushrooms and spinach followed by the softer parsley and yogurt.

Nutritional Facts (per serving):

- Calories: 100

- Vitamin D: 25 IU (6% Daily Value)

- Vitamin K: 200mcg (167% Daily Value)

- Potassium: 400mg (11% Daily Value)

TIPs:

- Substitute portobello mushrooms for a slightly stronger flavor.

- If the juice is too savory, add a squeeze of lemon or a few slices of apple for a touch of sweetness.

- This juice is best enjoyed immediately for optimal flavor and nutrient content.

Anti-inflammatory Juices for Bone Health: Soothing Your Body, Strengthening Your Bones

Chronic inflammation can negatively impact bone health. This chapter explores the power of anti-inflammatory juices, featuring delicious recipes rich in fruits and vegetables known for their anti-inflammatory properties. These vibrant juices can help combat inflammation and create a supportive environment for strong bones.

Berry Anti-Oxidation Blend

This antioxidant powerhouse juice bursts with delicious berries and a touch of pomegranate for a refreshing and anti-inflammatory boost.

Ingredients:

- 1 cup Blueberries (frozen)
- 1 cup Raspberries (frozen)
- 1/2 cup Cherries (pitted, frozen)
- 1/4 cup Pomegranate Seeds (fresh or frozen)

Instructions:

- Wash and freeze the berries and pomegranate seeds for at least 30 minutes before juicing.
- Add all Ingredients to your juicer, starting with the harder pomegranate seeds followed by the softer berries.

Nutritional Facts (per serving):

- Calories: 120
- Vitamin C: 200% Daily Value
- Manganese: 2mg (100% Daily Value)
- Fiber: 4 grams (16% Daily Value)

TIPs:

- Substitute other berries like strawberries or blackberries for a flavor variation.
- If the juice is too tart, add a squeeze of lime or a few slices of banana for a touch of sweetness.
- This juice is best enjoyed immediately for optimal flavor and nutrient content.

Green Detox Delight

This vibrant green juice is packed with leafy greens and refreshing vegetables for a detoxifying and anti-inflammatory boost.

Ingredients:

- 2 cups Spinach (fresh)
- 1 cup Kale (chopped)
- 1 Cucumber (peeled, chopped)
- 2 stalks Celery (chopped)

Instructions:

- Wash and chop all **Ingredient**s.
- Feed the **Ingredient**s into your juicer, starting with the harder vegetables (celery and cucumber) followed by the softer greens (spinach and kale).

Nutritional Facts (per serving):

- Calories: 50
- Vitamin K: 500mcg (417% Daily Value)
- Vitamin A: 150% Daily Value
- Folate: 100mcg (25% Daily Value)

TIPs:

- This juice can be slightly bitter due to the kale. If desired, add a few slices of apple or pear for a touch of sweetness.
- Leftover pulp can be added to smoothies, soups, or used in baking for a nutritional boost.

Turmeric Powerhouse

This vibrant orange juice harnesses the anti-inflammatory power of turmeric and ginger, with a touch of sweetness from apple and carrots.

Ingredients:

- 1 inch Turmeric Root (peeled, chopped)
- 1 inch Ginger Root (peeled, chopped)
- 2 Carrots (chopped)
- 1 Apple (chopped)

Instructions:

- Wash and chop all **Ingredient**s.
- Start by juicing the turmeric and ginger root (they are the most fibrous).
- Then, juice the carrots and apple.

Nutritional Facts (per serving):

- Calories: 150
- Vitamin A: 200% Daily Value
- Vitamin C: 20% Daily Value

- Manganese: 1.5mg (75% Daily Value)

TIPs:

- Fresh turmeric root can have a strong flavor. Start with a small amount and adjust to your preference.

- You can substitute pre-ground turmeric powder (½ teaspoon) for the fresh root, but fresh offers a more concentrated source of beneficial curcumin.

- This juice is best enjoyed immediately for optimal flavor and nutrient content.

CHAPTER 6

CUSTOMIZING YOUR JUICING JOURNEY: A PERSONALIZED APPROACH TO BONE HEALTH

While the previous chapters offered a foundation for juicing for bone health, your journey is unique. This chapter explores strategies for customizing your juicing routine to address dietary restrictions, manage other health conditions alongside osteoporosis, and create a personalized plan that fits your lifestyle.

Addressing Dietary Restrictions:

- ✓ **Vegetarian:** Load up on calcium-rich leafy greens, calcium-fortified plant milks, and tofu. Explore recipes featuring vegetables like broccoli and cauliflower, both excellent sources of bone-building vitamin K.

- ✓ **Vegan:** Similar to vegetarians, vegans can leverage calcium-rich vegetables and fortified plant milks. Opt for recipes with nuts and seeds, which offer additional calcium and protein. Consider adding a vegan calcium supplement after consulting with your doctor.

✓ **Dairy-Free:** Choose calcium-fortified plant milks and yogurt alternatives. Leafy greens, nuts, seeds, and fortified tofu are excellent sources of calcium for a dairy-free juicing plan.

Managing Other Health Conditions alongside Osteoporosis:

✓ **Diabetes:** Focus on low-glycemic fruits and vegetables in your juicing recipes. Sweeteners like stevia can be used sparingly if needed. Monitor your blood sugar levels and consult with your doctor to ensure juicing aligns with your diabetes management plan.

✓ **Kidney Disease:** Consult your doctor before starting any new dietary regimen, including juicing. Potassium and phosphorus content in certain fruits and vegetables may need to be monitored for individuals with kidney disease.

✓ **Digestive Issues:** Juicing can be a beneficial way to ensure nutrient absorption for those with digestive challenges. However, some individuals may experience digestive discomfort from the high fiber content of certain fruits and vegetables. Experiment with different combinations and consult a doctor or registered dietitian for personalized advice.

Creating a Personalized Juicing Plan:

- ✓ **Consider your taste preferences:** Experiment with different fruits and vegetables to find combinations you enjoy. This will ensure you're more likely to stick with your juicing routine.

- ✓ **Address your nutritional needs:** Focus on incorporating calcium-rich, Vitamin D rich, and anti-inflammatory fruits and vegetables into your juicing plan.

- ✓ **Start slow:** Begin with one or two juices per day and gradually increase as your body adjusts.

- ✓ **Variety is key:** Don't limit yourself to a few recipes. Explore different flavor combinations and **Ingredient**s to keep your juicing journey interesting.

- ✓ **Listen to your body:** Pay attention to how your body feels after consuming juices. Adjust your plan based on any digestive issues or blood sugar fluctuations.

- ✓ **Juicing is a supplement, not a replacement:** Maintain a balanced diet rich in whole fruits and vegetables alongside your juicing routine.

The road to stronger bones is paved with a combination of a healthy lifestyle, a balanced diet, and potentially medical treatment. Juicing can be a powerful tool in your bone health toolbox, offering a convenient and delicious way to incorporate essential nutrients and support your body's natural ability to build and maintain strong bones.

PART 3: LIVING WELL WITH OSTEOPOROSIS

CHAPTER 7

BEYOND JUICING: ESSENTIAL LIFESTYLE STRATEGIES FOR BONE HEALTH

While juicing offers a concentrated dose of bone-building nutrients, it's just one piece of the puzzle. A comprehensive approach to bone health requires a combination of dietary strategies, regular exercise, stress management, and a supportive network. This chapter delves into essential lifestyle strategies that complement your juicing journey and empower you to build strong, resilient bones.

The Importance of Exercise for Bone Density:

Just like muscles, bones respond to stress by becoming stronger. Regular exercise, particularly weight-bearing and resistance training, plays a crucial role in maintaining bone density and reducing the risk of fractures. Here's why exercise matters:

- **Stimulates bone formation:** Weight-bearing exercises like walking, jogging, dancing, and stair climbing put stress on bones, prompting the body to build new bone tissue.

- **Improves muscle strength:** Strong muscles support and stabilize bones, reducing the risk of falls and fractures.

- **Enhances balance and coordination:** Exercise helps improve balance and coordination, which can prevent falls, a significant risk factor for bone fractures.

Here are some TIPs for incorporating exercise into your bone health routine:

- **Aim for at least 30 minutes of moderate-intensity weight-bearing exercise most days of the week.** This could include brisk walking, jogging, dancing, or strength training exercises that target major muscle groups.

- **Find activities you enjoy:** You're more likely to stick with an exercise routine if you find it fun and engaging. Explore different activities like group fitness classes, swimming, yoga, or Pilates.

- **Start slowly and gradually increase intensity and duration.** Listen to your body and gradually increase the intensity and duration of your workouts to avoid injuries.

- **Consult with a doctor or physical therapist** before starting any new exercise program, especially if you have any underlying health conditions.

Maintaining a Balanced Diet for Overall Wellbeing:

While juicing provides a concentrated source of nutrients, it lacks the fiber content found in whole fruits and vegetables. A balanced diet rich in a variety of essential nutrients is crucial for overall health and bone health. Here are some dietary components to prioritize:

- ✓ **Calcium:** Aim for a daily intake of 1000mg for adults (increased to 1200mg for women over 50 and men over 70). Include calcium-rich foods like dairy products (if tolerated), leafy greens, fortified plant-based milks, tofu, and salmon.
- ✓ **Vitamin D:** Vitamin D helps with calcium absorption. Aim for 600 IU daily for adults. Include fatty fish, eggs, and fortified foods like milk and cereals in your diet. Sunlight exposure can also contribute to Vitamin D production, but consult your doctor for safe sun exposure guidelines.

- ✓ **Protein:** Protein is essential for building and maintaining bone tissue. Include lean protein sources like chicken, fish, beans, lentils, and nuts in your diet.
- ✓ **Fruits and Vegetables:** These offer a wealth of vitamins, minerals, and antioxidants that support overall health and bone health. Aim for a variety of colorful fruits and vegetables every day.

Building a Support System and Managing Stress:

Chronic stress can negatively impact bone health. Building a strong support system and practicing stress management techniques can play a vital role in your overall well-being and contribute to bone health. Here are some strategies to consider:

- ✓ **Connect with loved ones:** Having supportive relationships can help you cope with stress and provide emotional encouragement.
- ✓ **Join a support group:** Connecting with others who understand the challenges of osteoporosis can be invaluable.

- ✓ **Practice relaxation techniques:** Activities like meditation, yoga, deep breathing exercises, and spending time in nature can help manage stress and promote relaxation.
- ✓ **Seek professional help:** If you're struggling to manage stress, consider seeking help from a therapist or counselor.
- ✓ your quality of life and contribute to your bone health journey.

Juicing, combined with a balanced diet, regular exercise, stress management, and a supportive network, can empower you to take charge of your bone health. By incorporating these essential lifestyle strategies, you can create a holistic approach to building strong, resilient bones and promoting overall well-being.

CHAPTER 8

LONG-TERM MANAGEMENT OF OSTEOPOROSIS: A JOURNEY OF STRENGTH AND RESILIENCE

Osteoporosis is a chronic condition, but it doesn't have to define your life. With a proactive approach and ongoing collaboration with your doctor, you can effectively manage your osteoporosis and build a strong foundation for a healthy future. This chapter delves into the importance of long-term management strategies, explores treatment options, and emphasizes the power of healthy habits.

Working with Your Doctor: Monitoring Progress and Treatment Options

Regular communication and follow-up with your doctor are crucial for successful osteoporosis management. Here's what to expect:

✓ **Bone Density Scans (DXA scans):** These scans measure bone mineral density and monitor changes over time, helping your doctor assess treatment effectiveness and adjust strategies as needed.

✓ **Reviewing Treatment Options:** Your doctor will work with you to develop a personalized treatment plan based on your individual needs and medical history. Treatment options may include:

✓ **Medication:** Bisphosphonates, denosumab, and other medications can help slow bone loss and increase bone density.

✓ **Hormone Replacement Therapy (HRT):** For women experiencing menopause-related bone loss, HRT may be an option to consider.

✓ **Pain Management:** If you experience pain due to osteoporosis, your doctor can recommend medication and non-medicinal pain management strategies.

✓ **Building Healthy Habits for a Strong Future:**

✓ Beyond medications and doctor visits, incorporating healthy habits into your daily life is fundamental for long-term bone health management. Here are some key strategies to focus on:

✓ **Maintain a Balanced Diet:** As discussed previously, a diet rich in calcium, Vitamin D, protein, fruits, and vegetables provides the essential nutrients your bones need to thrive.

✓ **Regular Exercise:** Weight-bearing and resistance exercises remain vital for stimulating bone formation and maintaining bone density. Aim for at least 30 minutes of moderate-intensity exercise most days of the week.

✓ **Fall Prevention:** Falls are a major risk factor for fractures in individuals with osteoporosis. Implement fall prevention measures at home, such as improving lighting, removing tripping hazards, and installing grab bars in bathrooms.

✓ **Maintain a Healthy Weight:** Being overweight or obese can put additional stress on your bones. Work with your doctor to establish a healthy weight management plan if needed.

✓ **Don't Smoke and Limit Alcohol Consumption:** Smoking and excessive alcohol intake can weaken bones and hinder calcium absorption. Quitting smoking and limiting alcohol consumption are crucial for bone health.

✓ **Get Enough Sleep:** Adequate sleep is essential for overall health, including bone health. Aim for 7-8 hours of quality sleep each night.

69 | Juicing for Osteoporosis

CHAPTER 9

STAYING MOTIVATED AND INSPIRED ON YOUR JUICING JOURNEY: CULTIVATING LONG-TERM COMMITMENT

Embarking on a juicing journey for bone health is a positive step towards a stronger you. However, like any health initiative, maintaining motivation and staying on track can be challenging. This chapter equips you with strategies to overcome obstacles, celebrate successes, and cultivate a lasting love for healthy living.

Overcoming Challenges and Staying on Track:

- ✓ **Set Realistic Goals:** Don't aim for perfection. Start with achievable goals, like juicing twice a week, and gradually increase frequency as you establish a routine.

- ✓ **Plan and Prep:** Having **Ingredient**s prepped in advance saves time and reduces the temptation to skip juicing due to busy schedules.

- ✓ **Batch Prep Juices:** If time is a constraint, consider making larger batches of juice and storing them in airtight containers in the refrigerator for up to 24 hours.

- ✓ **Find a Juicing Buddy:** Enlist a friend or family member to join your juicing journey. Sharing experiences and offering support can boost motivation.

- ✓ **Explore New Recipes:** Experiment with different flavors and **Ingredient**s to keep your juicing routine exciting.

- ✓ **Embrace Imperfections:** Don't let occasional missed juicing days derail your progress. Get back on track and celebrate your commitment most of the time.

Celebrating Successes and Finding Joy in Healthy Living:

- ✓ **Track Your Progress:** Monitor your energy levels, bone density (through doctor-recommended scans), and overall well-being. Celebrate improvements, no matter how small.

✓ **Focus on How You Feel:** Pay attention to the positive changes in your body, like increased energy or improved digestion. This positive reinforcement can fuel motivation.

✓ **Connect the Dots:** Recognize how juicing contributes to your overall health goals. Feeling good empowers you to continue your juicing journey.

✓ **Make it Fun:** Explore new flavor combinations, decorate your juice glasses, or play upbeat music while juicing.

✓ **Find Joy in the Process:** View juicing as a form of self-care and a celebration of your commitment to a healthy lifestyle.

Beyond Juicing: Embracing a Holistic Approach to Health

While juicing offers a concentrated dose of nutrients, it's just one piece of the healthy living puzzle. Consider these additional strategies to integrate into your lifestyle:

✓ **Explore Healthy Cooking:** Learn to prepare delicious and nutritious meals that complement your juicing routine.

✓ **Prioritize Sleep:** Aim for 7-8 hours of quality sleep each night for optimal physical and mental health.

✓ **Manage Stress:** Practice relaxation techniques like meditation, yoga, or deep breathing exercises to manage stress and promote overall well-being.

✓ **Spend Time in Nature:** Immersing yourself in nature offers numerous health benefits, including improved mood and stress reduction.

Juicing can be a powerful tool for supporting bone health and a gateway to a healthier you. By incorporating the strategies outlined

BONUS

JUICING RECIPES FOR BONE HEALTH: BUILDING STRONG BONES, ONE SIP AT A TIME

Calcium-Rich Juices:

Green Powerhouse Juice (serves 1)

Ingredients:

- 2 cups kale (chopped),
- 1 cup spinach (fresh),
- 2 stalks celery (chopped), 1 orange (peeled)

Instructions:

- Wash and chop all Ingredients.
- Feed Ingredients into your juicer, starting with the harder vegetables followed by the softer greens.

Nutritional Facts:

- Calories: 50, Calcium: 200mg (16% Daily Value), Vitamin C: 120% Daily Value, Vitamin K: 500mcg (417% Daily Value)

TIP:

- This juice can be slightly bitter due to the kale.

- Add a few slices of apple or pear for a touch of sweetness.

- Leftover pulp can be added to smoothies, soups, or used in baking for a nutritional boost.

Tropical Calcium Blast (serves 1)

Ingredients:

- 1 cup mango (chopped), 1 cup pineapple (chopped), ½ banana (frozen), ½ cup plain yogurt (unsweetened),

- Add all ingredients to your juicer, starting with the frozen banana followed by the softer fruits and yogurt.

Instructions:

- Wash, chop, and freeze the banana for at least 30 minutes before juicing.

- Wash and chop the mango and pineapple.
- Add all ingredients to your juicer, starting with the frozen banana followed by the softer fruits and yogurt

Nutritional Facts:

- Calories: 200, Calcium: 250mg (20% Daily Value), Vitamin C: 200% Daily Value, Potassium: 400mg (11% Daily Value)

TIP:

- Substitute unsweetened Greek yogurt for a
- thicker consistency.
- If the juice is too sweet, add a squeeze of lime or lemon for a touch of tartness.

Creamy Berry Boost (serves 1)

Ingredients:

- 1 cup strawberries (frozen),
- 1 cup blueberries (frozen),
- ½ cup almond milk (unsweetened),
- ¼ cup plain yogurt (unsweetened)

Instructions:

- Wash and freeze the berries for at least 30 minutes before juicing.
- Add all Ingredients to your juicer, starting with the frozen berries followed by the yogurt and almond milk.

Nutritional Facts:

- Calories: 150, Calcium: 200mg (16% Daily Value), Vitamin C: 150% Daily Value, Manganese: 1.5mg (75% Daily Value)

TIP:

- Substitute other berries like raspberries or blackberries for a flavor variation.
- If the juice is too thick, add a little more almond milk for a thinner consistency.

Vitamin D Rich Juices:

Sunshine Citrus Splash (serves 1)

Ingredients:

- 2 oranges (peeled),
- 1 grapefruit (peeled, halved),

- 1 carrot (chopped)

Instructions:

- Wash and chop the carrot.

- Peel the oranges and grapefruit, removing any white pith if desired for a less bitter taste.

- Feed the Ingredients into your juicer, starting with the harder carrot followed by the softer citrus fruits.

Nutritional Facts:

- CalAories: 100, Vitamin D: 20 IU (5% Daily Value), Vitamin C: 200% Daily Value, Beta-Carotene: 10,000 IU (200% Daily Value)

TIP:

- This juice can be slightly tart due to the grapefruit.

- Add a squeeze of lime or a few slices of apple for a touch of sweetness.

- Leftover carrot pulp can be used in soups, stews, or baking recipes.

Tropical D Delight (serves 1)

Ingredients:

- 1 cup mango (chopped),
- 1 cup pineapple (chopped),
- ½ cup papaya (chopped)

Instructions:

- Wash and chop all Ingredients.
- Feed the Ingredients into your juicer, starting with the harder fruits (papaya) followed by the softer ones (mango and pineapple).

Nutritional Facts:

- Calories: 150, Vitamin D: 15 IU (4% Daily Value), Vitamin C: 250% Daily Value, Manganese: 1mg (50% Daily Value)

TIP:

- Substitute other tropical fruits like guava or passion fruit for a flavor variation.

Creamy Mushroom Magic (serves 1)

Ingredients:

- 1 cup white mushrooms (sliced),
- 1 cup spinach (fresh),

- ¼ cup parsley (fresh),
- ½ cup plain yogurt (unsweetened)

Instructions:

- Wash and slice the mushrooms.
- Wash the spinach and parsley.
- Add all Ingredients to your juicer, starting with the harder mushrooms and spinach followed by the softer parsley and yogurt.

Nutritional Facts:

- Calories: 100, Vitamin D: 25 IU (6% Daily Value), Vitamin K: 200mcg (167% Daily Value), Potassium: 400mg (11% Daily Value)

TIP:

- Substitute portobello mushrooms for a slightly stronger flavor.
- If the juice is too savory, add a squeeze of lemon or a few slices of apple for a touch of sweetness.
- This juice is best enjoyed immediately for optimal flavor and nutrient content.

Sunshine on a Cloud (serves 1)

Ingredients:

- 1 cup cantaloupe (chopped),
- ½ cup orange (peeled),
- ¼ cup fortified plant-based milk (vitamin D enriched)

Instructions:

- Wash and chop the cantaloupe and orange.
- Add all Ingredients to your juicer, starting with the harder orange followed by the softer cantaloupe and milk.

Nutritional Facts:

- Calories: 120, Vitamin D: 100 IU (25% Daily Value) (from fortified milk), Vitamin C: 100% Daily Value, Potassium: 300mg (8% Daily Value)

TIP:

- Substitute honeydew melon for cantaloupe for a slightly different flavor.
- Choose a fortified plant-based milk with at least 100 IU of Vitamin D per serving.
-

Anti-inflammatory Juices:

Berry Anti-Oxidation Blend (serves 1)

Ingredients:

- 1 cup blueberries (frozen),
- 1 cup raspberries (frozen),
- 1/2 cup cherries (pitted, frozen),
- 1/4 cup pomegranate seeds (fresh or frozen)

Instructions:

- Wash and freeze the berries and pomegranate seeds for at least 30 minutes before juicing.
- Add all Ingredients to your juicer, starting with the harder pomegranate seeds followed by the softer berries.

Nutritional Facts:

- Calories: 120, Vitamin C: 200% Daily Value, Manganese: 2mg (100% Daily Value), Fiber: 4 grams (16% Daily Value)

TIP:

- Substitute other berries like strawberries or blackberries for a flavor variation.

- If the juice is too tart, add a squeeze of lime or a few slices of banana for a touch of sweetness.

- This juice is best enjoyed immediately for optimal flavor and nutrient content.

Green Detox Delight (serves 1)

Ingredients:

- 2 cups spinach (fresh),

- 1 cup kale (chopped),

- 1 cucumber (peeled, chopped),

- 2 stalks celery (chopped)

Instructions:

- Wash and chop all Ingredients.

- Feed the Ingredients into your juicer, starting with the harder vegetables (celery and cucumber) followed by the softer greens (spinach and kale).

Nutritional Facts:

- Calories: 50, Vitamin K: 500mcg (417% Daily Value), Vitamin A: 150% Daily Value, Folate: 100mcg (25% Daily Value)

TIP:

- This juice can be slightly bitter due to the kale.
- Add a few slices of apple or pear for a touch of sweetness.
- Leftover pulp can be added to smoothies, soups, or used in baking for a nutritional boost.

Turmeric Powerhouse (serves 1)

Ingredients:

- 1 inch turmeric root (peeled, chopped),
- 1 inch ginger root (peeled, chopped),
- 2 carrots (chopped), 1 apple (chopped)

Instructions:

- Wash and chop all Ingredients. Start by juicing the turmeric and ginger root (they are the most fibrous).
- Then, juice the carrots and apple.

Nutritional Facts:

- Calories: 150, Vitamin A: 200% Daily Value, Vitamin C: 20% Daily Value, Manganese: 1.5mg (75% Daily Value)

TIP:

- Fresh turmeric root can have a strong flavor. Start with a small amount and adjust to your preference.

- You can substitute pre-ground turmeric powder (½ teaspoon) for the fresh root, but fresh offers a more concentrated source of beneficial curcumin.

- This juice is best enjoyed immediately for optimal flavor and nutrient content.

Additional Bone-Supporting Juices:

Beetroot Power Punch (serves 1)

Ingredients:

- 1 medium beet (peeled, chopped), 1 carrot (chopped), 1 apple (chopped), ½ lemon (peeled)

Instructions:

- Wash, peel, and chop all Ingredients.
- Start by juicing the beet (it's the hardest) followed by the carrot, apple, and lemon.

Nutritional Facts:

- Calories: 150, Vitamin C: 30% Daily Value, Folate: 50mcg (13% Daily Value), Manganese: 0.5mg (3% Daily Value)

TIP:

- Beets can stain! Wear gloves while handling them and be mindful when cleaning your juicer.

- The juice can be strong flavored. Start with a smaller amount of beet and adjust to your preference.

Green Goddess (serves 1)

Ingredients:

- 2 cups romaine lettuce (chopped),
- 1 cup broccoli florets,
- ½ cucumber (peeled, chopped),
- 1 kiwi fruit
- (peeled)

Instructions:

- Wash and chop all Ingredients. Start by juicing the harder broccoli florets and cucumber followed by the softer romaine lettuce and kiwi.

Nutritional Facts:

- Calories: 80, Vitamin K: 150mcg (125% Daily Value), Vitamin C: 100% Daily Value, Folate: 30mcg (8% Daily Value)

TIP:

- Broccoli can be slightly bitter.

- Add a few slices of apple or pear for a touch of sweetness.

Sunshine on a Stick (serves 1)

Ingredients:

- 1 cup celery (chopped),

- 1 carrot (chopped),

- 1 orange (peeled),

- ½ cup pineapple (chopped)

Instructions:

- Wash and chop all Ingredients.

- Start by juicing the harder celery and carrot followed by the softer orange and pineapple.

Nutritional Facts:

- Calories: 120, Vitamin C: 200% Daily Value, Vitamin A: 150% Daily Value, Potassium: 400mg (11% Daily Value)

TIP:

- Substitute other citrus fruits like grapefruit or tangerines for a flavor variation.

Berry Blast (serves 1)

Ingredients:

- 1 cup strawberries (frozen),
- 1 cup blueberries (frozen),
- 1 banana (frozen),
- ½ cup plain yogurt (unsweetened)

Instructions:

- Wash and freeze the berries and banana for at least 30 minutes before juicing.
- Add all Ingredients to your juicer, starting with the frozen banana and berries followed by the yogurt.

Nutritional Facts:

- Calories: 250, Calcium: 125mg (10% Daily Value), Vitamin C: 150% Daily Value, Manganese: 1mg (50% Daily Value)

TIP:

- Substitute other berries like raspberries or blackberries for a flavor variation. For a thicker consistency, use Greek yogurt.

Tropical Sunshine (serves 1)

Ingredients:

- 1 cup mango (chopped),
- ½ cup pineapple (chopped),
- ½ cup papaya (chopped),
- ½ lime (peeled)

Instructions:

- Wash and chop all Ingredients.
- Start by juicing the lime (it's the hardest) followed by the softer fruits.

Nutritional Facts

- Calories: 180, Vitamin C: 200% Daily Value, Manganese: 1mg (50% Daily Value), Fiber: 3 grams (12% Daily Value)

TIP:

- Substitute other tropical fruits like guava or passion fruit for a flavor variation.

Protein-Rich Juices

Berry Protein Boost (serves 1)

Ingredients:

- 1 cup mixed berries (frozen - strawberries, blueberries, raspberries)
- ½ banana (frozen)
- 1 scoop protein powder (unflavored or berry flavored)
- ½ cup plain yogurt (unsweetened)

Instructions:

- Wash and freeze the berries and banana for at least 30 minutes before juicing.

- Add all Ingredients to your juicer, starting with the frozen banana and berries followed by the protein powder and yogurt.

- Blend all Ingredients well after juicing for a smoother consistency.

Nutritional Facts

- (depending on protein powder used): Calories: 250, Protein: 20g, Calcium: 125mg (10% Daily Value), Vitamin C: 150% Daily Value

TIP:

- Choose a protein powder that complements the berry flavor. For a thicker consistency, use Greek yogurt.

Green Veggie & Hemp Power (serves 1)

Ingredients:

- 2 cups spinach (fresh)
- 1 cup cucumber (peeled, chopped)
- 1 celery stalk (chopped)
- 1 tablespoon hemp seeds

Instructions:

- Wash and chop all Ingredients.
- Add all Ingredients to your juicer, starting with the harder cucumber and celery followed by the softer spinach and hemp seeds.
- Pulse the juicer a few times to incorporate the hemp seeds effectively.

Nutritional Facts:

- Calories: 80, Protein: 3g (6% Daily Value), Vitamin K: 300mcg (250% Daily Value), Manganese: 1mg (50% Daily Value)

TIP:

- Hemp seeds offer a good source of plant-based protein and healthy fats.
- You can substitute ground flaxseeds for a similar nutritional profile.

Tropical Protein Paradise (serves 1)

Ingredients:

- 1 cup mango (chopped)
- ½ cup pineapple (chopped)
- ½ cup papaya (chopped)
- 1 scoop collagen peptide powder (unflavored or fruit flavored)

Instructions:

- Wash and chop all Ingredients.
- Mix the collagen peptide powder well with a little water before adding it to the juicer to avoid clumping.
- Add all Ingredients to your juicer, starting with the harder fruits followed by the collagen peptide powder.

Nutritional Facts

- (depending on collagen peptide powder used): Calories: 200,
- Protein: 10g (20% Daily Value),
- Vitamin C: 200% Daily Value,
- Manganese: 1mg (50% Daily Value)

TIP:

- Collagen peptides can support bone health and joint health.

- Choose a flavorless powder or one that complements the tropical fruits.

CONCLUSION

A FINAL WORD: EMPOWERING YOURSELF THROUGH JUICING AND BEYOND

Osteoporosis may present challenges, but it doesn't have to define your future. You hold the power to take charge of your bone health and build a strong foundation for a vibrant life. Juicing offers a delicious and convenient way to incorporate essential bone-building nutrients into your daily routine.

This journey is more than just about juicing; it's about empowerment. By taking an active role in your health, exploring healthy recipes, and incorporating juicing into a holistic lifestyle, you can:

➢ **Nourish your body with essential nutrients** to support strong bones and overall well-being.

➢ **Experience a renewed sense of vitality and energy.**

- ➢ **Cultivate a positive mindset** focused on self-care and proactive health management.
- ➢ **Inspire others** to embrace healthy habits and prioritize their well-being.